Canning and Preserving

CANNING & PRESERVING

Making Your Food Last
While It's Good!

Second Edition

Edgar Walker

© 2016

Canning and Preserving
©Copyright 2016

Disclaimer

incorporate and apply all the information provided. Although the writer will make his best effort share her insights, the topic in question is a complex one, and each person needs a different timeframe to fully incorporate new information. Neither this book, nor any of the author's books constitute a promise that the reader will learn anything within a certain timeframe.

Canning and Preserving

Table of Content

Introduction

Since the very beginning, people have dependably searched for approaches to sustain a steady nourishment supply. One of the ways that individuals do this is by purchasing canned sustenance or by canning their own produced such as the fruits and vegetables. This keeps up the freshness that is frequently just caught through chilling and solidifying, and keeps the food delicate and chewable, rather than making it hard and difficult to chew like how drying the food always does.

The historical backdrop of canning truly starts with Napoleon as he searched for approaches to nourish his huge armed forces as they walked crosswise over Europe. As time proceeded onward, canning got to be distinctly computerized, yet exceptionally unregulated, taking into consideration high measures of defilement that made a few people debilitated and killed some too. Even so, various individuals additionally learned and did canning at home. A large number of them are willing to discover approaches to save money on their own nourishment costs and to extend whatever they developed in their own particular garden to last the whole year. With an extensively more directed canning industry, the quantity of issues that emerged toward the start of industrialized canning has turned out to be significantly more secure and is a standout amongst the most usually sold things in markets today.

In any case, if you're fascinated with doing canning at home, don't stress. There are a lot of areas for you to go for procedures and general aid. Although, there are some exceptionally strict rules that you have to follow with a specific end goal to ensure that you and your family are safe from a bug that figured out how to get into the container when you were canning. Be that as it may, never allow this to discourage you from trying a new venture like this.

Canning is a decent route for extending vegetables into the winter, particularly when coolers aren't accessible. If done appropriately, canning is a sealed shut and safe approach to keep bugs and sicknesses out of your garden-fresh leafy foods and whatever else that you might need to can, similar to sauces of different sorts or sticks or jams. This book will walk you through the general procedure of canning. In the end, you can go out and investigate the domain of canning all alone and conceivably join two or three online groups that can and give you direction in a way that a book can't give.

History of Canning and Preserving

People have constantly discovered approaches to sustain the freshness of the food, whether it's through drying, pickling, smoking, or aging. In any case, the issue with every one of those strategies for safeguarding is that there's no real way to keep the nourishment in a new state. Chilling crisp foods grown from the ground (fruits and vegetables) was impossible until coolers arrived. This is the only other option that sustenance is kept genuinely new and defended from rotting causes.

Before the 1700s, canning just didn't exist. Individuals had realized that air frequently causes illnesses and parasites that would make the food turn sour, however, they hadn't exactly discovered how to save and keep it far from the air. The nearest approach they had come was cooking meat and after that concealing it under a layer of fat, which would just protect the meat for a brief timeframe.

In spite of the fact that Pasteur wasn't able to reach fifty more years to clarify the presence of microorganisms, individuals had started to understand that expelling air from safeguarded foods would amplify the time span of usability, though they were not exactly sure how to perfectly do it yet.

In the late 1700s, France was at war and expected to figure out how to nourish the armed force that was presently spread over the world. Willing to figure out how to nourish troops, the French government (through the French Directory) offered a twelve thousand franc prize through the Society for the Encouragement of Industry for a leap forward path in the sustaining the nutrients on the food in 1795. By 1809, Napoleon was sovereign of France and the armed forces were much hungrier as they walked crosswise Europe.

Nicolas Appert, a confectioner and a culinary specialist for the honorability, responded to the call and started trying different things about food conservation. Taking the most grounded water/air proof compartments that he had permission to (champagne bottles), Appert figured out how to fruitfully seal the containers by combining cheddar and lime while utilizing heat to help the fixing procedure. He demonstrated it by safeguarding soups, juices, and a few vegetables. The fundamental way that his procedure worked was to place food in the champagne jugs and stuck caps after that before covering them with wax. When they were totally covered, the jugs were wrapped in canvas and boiled.

By 1803, he had advanced to safeguarding vegetables, organic product, meat, dairy, and fish, and had let the food out to be tried on the high oceans with the French Navy. After a year, Appert started to safeguard meat in tin jars by fastening the tops on, if the tins didn't swell, then they were viewed as protected and sold for long haul stockpiling and usage. In 1809, Appert was granted the twelve thousand franc prize, in the condition that he paid to distribute the strategy that he used to protect his food. He did that a year later, emancipating The Art of Preserving, for Several Years, All Animal and Vegetable Substances. The procedure that Appert utilized was astonishing, not just in light of the fact that Pasteur wouldn't have the chance to appear and clarify why the procedure worked so well for an additional fifty years, but since the can opener wouldn't be created for an additional thirty years. Troopers would frequently wound the jars with pikes to open them or they would be etched open. Once he'd won the prize, Appert would keep on working on his strategy, however the industrial facilities he utilized, though inventive, were unrewarding and he kicked the bucket poor in 1841.

Despite the fact that Appert was the master of canning in France, the technique had immediately moved over the English Channel and was taken under the wing of Brian Donkin in 1812. Rather than utilizing glass, Donkin chose to utilize tin rather, which began the tin can industry. The procedure was at first moderate and work concentrated, as the tin jars were made by hand and the cooking procedure could take up to six hours. This likewise made the whole procedure to a great degree costly and drove the cost up a lot for a typical individual to truly manage. Once more, a lion's share of canned food was utilized for the British armed force and the Royal Navy, yet wayfarers would frequently bring canned foods with them in light of the fact that the conservation and little size made conveying the jars and containers perfect.

Amid the mid-1800s, canned products were viewed as a grown-up toy all over Europe, yet there were a few perils included, including the utilization of a lead patch to seal the jars. In any case, costs started to drop as new advancements joined the Industrial Revolution. The blast of the urban populace in Europe, alongside a more automated process that permitted a steel can to replace the tin jars, permitted the cooking time to drop from six hours to thirty minutes and make the item less expensive to make and purchase.

In the Americas, canning was additionally grabbing hold, spreading rapidly over the sea in 1812. Rather than utilizing a strong tin can, American makers utilized tin plated fashioned iron jars for safeguarding meats, clams, vegetables, and organic products. Amid the different wars, the interest for canned food rose exponentially, which would present various common laborers men to the food, and would likewise give organizations a chance to produce in mass before offering to a wide non-military personnel consumers. Before the end of the 1800s, and over the world, the market of canned goods had detonated in prominence and organizations endeavored to surpass each other by utilizing profoundly improved printed names, innovative foods, and modest costs.

The entry of World War I again expanded the request for canned goods that could survive the brutal states of the trenches and be transported securely. Toward the start of the war, officers were sustained low-quality canned nourishments. In any case, by 1916, confidence among troopers was low and in an effort to enhance it, armed forces started to receive improved food for their men, including canned sustenance that was a whole supper. In 1917, the French Army started conveying jars of coq au vin, vichyssoise, and beff bourguignon while the Italians ran with spaghetti Bolognese, ravioli, Pasta e fagioli, and Minestrone. As the war ended, the organizations that had figured out how to supply nourishment to the armed forces started to give better nature of canned foods to regular folks.

Canning and Preserving
Benefits and Dangers of Canning

When you can at home, there are various advantages that you may not know about, notwithstanding, there are likewise a few perils that you have to think about too. When you're canning, information is your best key to battling any threats that could emerge.

The greatest thing that you have to stress as far as canning, particularly home canning is Botulism. This wonder is brought on by the microbes clostridium botulinum. It's found in soil and will survive, develop, and make poisons in a fixed container of food, which will then make you greatly, tremendously debilitated. The poison that Botulism makes can influence your sensory system, which may incapacitate you and prompt to death. Nonetheless, there are a few signs that you can search for in canned goods (this additionally applies to store canned foods). In the event that the jug is releasing, protruding, or swollen, never

15

consume it, toss it out quickly. This likewise applies if the compartment is harmed, split, or for the most part looks anomalous. On the off chance that you open the holder and fluid or froth spurts out, dispose of it instantly and tidy up any spillage with dye. On the off chance that you investigate the holder and it notices terrible, is mildew covered, or stained, toss it out. By and large, on the off chance that you don't believe the can that you're going to open for any reason, don't. Toss it out. Somewhere around 1996 and 2014, there were two hundred and ten flare-ups of botulism brought about by nourishment. A hundred and forty-five of those flare-ups were brought about by home-arranged sustenances and forty-three originated from home-canned vegetables. Home-canning of vegetables are the most well-known reason for botulism in the United States. Be that as it may, a large portion of those cases are brought on by individuals overlooking canning directions, didn't utilize weight canners, disregarded the indications of the nourishment ruining, or simply didn't know the hazard from shamefully canned sustenances.

16

Realize what sort of nourishment you're canning. Nourishments that are low in sharpness (like corn, green beans, potatoes, fish, poultry, or meat) must be weight canned on the grounds that some other technique won't ensure you against botulism. In case you're uncertain with respect to regardless of whether a nourishment (especially vegetables) is high corrosive, the FDA gives a rundown of all pH values for sustenances on their site.

Many individuals get a kick out of the chance to utilize formulas passed on from era to era. Yet, with regards to canning, however, don't do that. Try not to utilize cookbooks or formulas that are obsolete with regards to canning. They might not have you get the sustenance sufficiently hot to slaughter any microscopic organisms or make them heat up the containers sufficiently long to seal them legitimately. Simply don't utilize obsolete formulas. It isn't ok for you or for the general population that you might give the jugs to as blessings.

There are many advantages to canning when it's set appropriately. Home-canned sustenances can last around 18 months on the rack, which makes them simple for you to use in the wake of a monotonous day to supplement your feast and ensure that you're getting enough products of the soil in your eating routine. This additionally implies if there's a characteristic fiasco or the like, canned sustenance gives a simple and prepared wellspring of moderately safe nourishment for you to eat that won't put you at danger of being defiled by anything.

Having canned nourishment additionally helps you amid terrible monetary circumstances. Economically canned nourishment can keep going for up to five years now and again, however regardless of the possibility that you home can, the measure of sustenance that you'll have to purchase is lessened in light of the fact that you have sustenance as of now stockpiled at home, all prepared to be utilized. Furthermore, on a tight spending plan, having canned nourishment ensures that despite everything you're getting the foods grown from the ground that you require when the cost of new products of the soil might be extensively more costly than you can stand to pay. (It would be ideal if you know, be that as it may, that canned leafy foods are not a perfect substitute for the genuine article.)

One of the many advantages of canning your own nourishment is that you can safeguard your gather or that of a nearby farmer's. In the wake of sitting tight for quite a long time for your garden to create natural product, you may get yourself overpowered. Canning will extend the reap to last more and diminish the measure of waste that may happen from a portion of the vegetables or natural product turning sour. A great deal of agriculturists additionally encounter this and will frequently offer a ton of their create for a shabby sum if the vibe overpowered by it. Investigating your neighborhood rancher's market and realizing what's in season will help you to arrange and get ready for a guard yield of specific vegetables or natural products.

Other than making a bond with nearby agriculturists, home canning is additionally eco-accommodating. The measure of waste that is made by home canning is impressively not as much as purchasing jars from the store. A great deal of the materials that are utilized as a part of home canning can be utilized quite a long time and you aren't tossing out various jars or covers that may wind up in nature. You're likewise eliminating the measure of gas and vitality that is utilized to transport the canned sustenance from the homestead to the production line then to the wholesaler and after that to the store. You're eliminating that much more on the off chance that you purchase from a rancher or utilize your own particular vegetables to can.

In spite of the fact that canning isn't the most beneficial approach to ensure you're getting your supplements, there are still various advantages to it. It's significantly more nutritious when you can the vegetables yourself since you know where it originated from and can control how much salt or sugar goes into it and, in the event that you choose to add any additives to the would, you be able to choose what amount goes in. An economically delivered container of canned products of the soil can contain a great deal of salt or sugar, in addition to you can't control the measure of or what sort of additives go into the can. In addition, many individuals say that home cooked suppers taste the best, and that is the same for home canned vegetables.

Individuals regularly make sticks and jams, which can then be given away as presents to loved ones. The measure of time and vitality that goes into canning can fill somebody's heart with joy, in addition, it will be delighted in over a drawn out stretch of time and will be enormously refreshing by the individuals who you offered it to. The way that the blessing was custom made may likewise make the individual feel like they're coming back to a more straightforward time, and they may appreciate that inclination.

There are various advantages that exceed the cons of canning. Learning is the most ideal approach to battle the perils of home canning and will likewise help to just teach you on the long convention of canning. Knowing the most ideal approach to securely safeguard nourishment by canning will help you to remain safe, and the signs that botulism might be available can likewise be effectively found in business jars too.

Materials Needed to Can

There are several key materials that will need to can keeping in mind the end goal to can well and securely. First off, will require jugs. Frequently, artisan jugs with a screw beat cover that works best. You can get them at any store in various sizes. When you purchase the jugs, they will accompany the rings (which you shouldn't have to supplant unless you lose one) and the top part of the top that goes down under the ring. The part that goes down under the ring should be supplanted each time you utilize that container to can in light of the fact that that is the part that seals the jug and "flies" to tell you this when the can is fixed. When it's been utilized, it must be supplanted, and you can discover substitutions in littler bundles. Other than what you're canning, these ought to be one of the not very many things that you'll have to purchase.

From your kitchen, you'll require a couple of tongs. The tongs will be utilized to force jugs and the top

23

parts from bubbling water. This is critical so you don't get singed before you truly start the canning procedure.

You're likewise going to require a wide mouth channel. Ensure that it doesn't surpass the extent of the jug's mouth since you'll be utilizing it to empty everything that you're canning into the container without spilling it all over the place. Having the pipe will genuinely decrease the likelihood that an expansive wreckage will happen and will help you ensure that you are working in a genuinely clean workspace. Regardless of the possibility that you feel that you can pour things splendidly, don't hazard it.

Various measuring containers will prove to be useful so you can spoon your canning blend into the jugs and ensure that they all have a similar measure of blend in it. This is essential so when you're bubbling or pressurizing the containers, they all get precisely the same of time. Having containers with changing sums in them won't give them a predictable cooking time and will compel you to

24

figure on regardless of whether the jugs are finished. Speculated, with regards to canning is awful.

This next instrument isn't a need, yet I would suggest it since it makes it more secure to expel jugs from the bubbling water and decreases the danger of a jug slipping from your grip and breaking. The apparatus would be a container lifter. It would seem that a couple of tongs, however has an exceptionally expansive, level handle with elastic wrapped tongs at the flip side that takes after the state of a container's head. This is the thing that you use to lower and raise the containers from the bubbling water when everything is fixed in. Despite the fact that not a need, it might give you less cerebral pains with regards to hauling everything out of the pots. On the off chance that you super would prefer not to get a container lifter, then ensure you have a couple of tongs with elastic toward one side or the other. That will protect you from the warmth and ensure that you won't get singed by the jugs as you lift them out.

Keeping in mind the end goal to have things to would, you're be able to going to require a nonreactive pot to cook the vegetables or the item that you're attempting to make for canning. The sort of pot truly doesn't make a difference. Simply utilize one of your standard clean cooking pots for setting up your item to can. Crude vegetables generally aren't canned, and you'll see this when you take a gander at formulas online for whatever you choose to can.

You're additionally going to require an expansive pot, similar to a stock pot, to really can in, particularly in case you're taking after the bubbling water technique. The pot should be sufficiently vast to hold the containers that you're canning and to ensure that the whole jug is shrouded in water. That will make the seal that you require. It additionally should be sufficiently tall to hold the jars or jugs when they're laying on a metal rack or a cloth.

Keeping in mind the end goal to can legitimately, the whole container or can needs boiling hot water streaming the distance around it, including around the base of the jugs. So as to ensure that the water is streaming around the jugs totally, they have to lay on a cloth or a rack or something to that affect. This will ensure that the majority of the bugs that might be in a can are slaughtered

One advantage of canning is that you don't generally need to purchase anything for it. The greater part of the stuff that you need is as of now in your home, and in the event that you do need to purchase anything, it's for the most part reusable from year to year. Additionally, a dominant part of what you require, you'll use all the time.

How to Can

With regards to canning, there are two strategies for you to consider. What technique you utilize will totally rely on upon what you're attempting to can because of the pH level of the sustenance. Nourishment that is viewed as acidic or a protect will for the most part run with a bubbling water shower; while sustenance that is low in causticity (like a lion's share of vegetables that aren't appropriately cured, poultry, fish, and meats) must be weight canned, which requires a particular weight cooker like contraption that will warm the containers to a specific temperature for a particular measure of time. This is vital in light of the fact that in spite of the fact that the microbes that causes botulism kicks the bucket at bubbling temperature, the spores that deliver the poisons can survive higher temperatures that the real microscopic organisms; also, they flourish in low-corrosive situations.

To start canning, discover a formula for whatever you need to can and read through it with a specific end goal to ensure that you have everything that you requirement for it. Additionally take note of the measure of time that you'll have to bubble or pressurize the jugs for, just so that you're mindful of how much time everything will take.

Once you've done that, take your tops and rings and place them in a little pot on the stove before covering them with water. Do a similar thing to the jugs (ensure they're put topsy turvy) in the stock pot, and turn the stove on. Heat the jugs to the point of boiling and the tops and rings to a slight stew. This will murder anything that might attempt to flourish in your jugs and will simply be a decent approach to clean everything without using cleanser on your containers and covers.

While everything bubbles, set up the formula that you're attempting to make. When you complete that, remove everything from the bubbling water utilizing your tongs and put them on a spotless towel that is on your counter. You can either give them a chance to air dry or utilize another wipe towel to get dry every one of the containers and covers.

At the point when everything is gotten dry, take your channel and measuring glasses and fill the jugs with your item. Contingent upon your formula, you'll need to leave a fourth of an inch to an a large portion of an inch of space between the surface of your item and the highest point of the container (which is additionally called headspace). Contingent upon the formula, you may need to delicately tap the container on the counter through the towel to ensure that all air bubbles have become out of the item. Ensure that you additionally wipe the lip of the container to ensure that everything is spotless and clear. On the off chance that the item is left on the lip of the container, then the jug covers may not seal accurately, which will imply that you can't store the item at all and should utilize it rapidly. At that point, apply the tops and screw the rings on to ensure that the tops don't move at all while they're being pressurized.

This is the place the two sorts of canning truly split. In case you're running with the weight can strategy, you'll simply need to put the jars in the weight cooker and time it painstakingly to ensure everything is pressurized and the covers are fixed legitimately. The formula will let you know for to what extent to keep the containers or jars in the pressurizer.

In case you're going will the bubbling strategy, you'll have to put the jars into the stockpot with the water as of now bubbling. Try to be to a great degree safe with this and utilize your container lifter to take them in and out. You may need to expel a portion of the water from the pot once you include the containers, so ensure you have a warmth evidence measuring glass available. Ensure that you additionally don't stack shakes on top of each other. Keep in mind, the water needs to course the whole jug, that is the reason you have the rack at the base of the container. Set your clock to the sum recorded on the formula, and ensure that you don't surpass that time.

When you take the jugs out, simply put them on the counter again and hold up. The jugs ought to begin pinging in the blink of an eye as the seals frame and the focal point of the tops give in to stamp the vacuum seal grabbing hold. After the jugs have cooled, take the rings off of the jugs, the covers ought to remain set up with the goal that you can check the seals. So as to do that, just handle the jug by the edge of the cover and lift it tenderly off the counter around an inch or two. In the event that the top doesn't move, you've made an effective seal and you can plan to store your canned products.

In the event that your containers didn't seal, then there were two or three things that may have happened. There could have been an item on the lip of the container, which may have made it inconceivable for the seal to really frame since there was something in the way. Another reason could be that the tops weren't stewed for a sufficiently long timeframe, the stewing serves to the sealant to mellow and it will have a considerable measure of inconvenience framing the seal if the sealant wasn't sufficiently delicate to shape a strong handle on the highest point of the jug. Ensure that when your item goes into the jug, it is to a great degree hot. There should be some warmth within the jug to make the vacuum as the air inside the container chills and pulls the cover off to make the ping.

In the event that you lost some of your item amid the bubbling or pressurizing process, then what may have happened is that the air bubbles that were caught in the container before endeavoring to seal the cover got away before the seal was framed advanced out amid the fixing procedure. It's nothing to truly stress over, simply attempt to ensure that your item is settled before you put it the stock pot or pressurizer for fixing.

In the event that you had a container that neglected to seal while you were canning, don't stress, the item is no doubt still great and you'll simply get the chance to appreciate it before any of the other fixed jars. When you utilize it, and on the off chance that you don't utilize every last bit of it without a moment's delay, ensure that you keep the opened jug in your fridge so it doesn't ruin. Ensure that you stamp the date on the greater part of your completely fixed jugs so as to ensure that you eat them inside the suggested time of eighteen months of the canning date. Anything after that date can get to be distinctly hazardous to devour and since you're not including numerous (assuming any) additives to the item, it can begin to really ruin.

Other Preservation Methods

Human culture wouldn't have advanced without figuring out how to save nourishment so as to help people to make due all through incline circumstances or through difficult winters. We've spent a dominant part of this book talking about canning and how to can so as to safeguard some of your new leafy foods. In any case, canning isn't the best way to safeguard organic products, vegetables, or meats, there are a great deal more ways that individuals can save their nourishment.

Bubbling – When you bubble nourishment, you possibly slaughter various conceivably destructive microbes. This strategy was found by Pasteur when it came to dairy. Thus, it is proceeded with today to protect a greater part of purchasers. This is likewise utilized with water to murder any terrible organisms that may exist. It is likewise utilized as a part of request to clean different materials utilized as a part of canning. There are various additive uses for bubbling, regularly the executing of little creatures that wreak devastation on the human body.

Internment – This is a sort of cellaring as it expels the light, mugginess, and temperature from various sustenances. It can likewise be utilized as a part of blend with the aging or salting strategies, and works best in soil that is dry and salty.

Cellaring – This technique is to a great degree simple for the vast majority to do at home in light of the fact that there are such a variety of thoughts and diverse routes for it to be finished. Everything is put away in a temperature-, light-, and stickiness controlled environment, which implies that it functions admirably with various diverse nourishments, similar to nuts, vegetables, aged sustenances, and dry-cured meats. A few strategies behind cellaring require reasonable hardware, while different techniques don't require any gear by any stretch of the imagination. To some degree, everyone can utilize the cellaring strategy to secure their nourishments.

Cooling – You may not understand it, but rather on the off chance that you have a fridge, you're utilizing the cooling technique at this moment to safeguard your new foods grown from the ground. Cooling nourishment moderates the development of different smaller scale life forms that causes the deterioration of new sustenance, similar to leafy foods.

Curing – This is a strategy that is to a great degree near pickling and uses a corrosive, salt, as well as nitrates and is most usually utilized on meats and fish. Advanced curing strategies have begun to lessen the measures of salt and nitrates in the meats, which implies that the nourishment then must be refrigerated or solidified to safeguard the last item. Nourishments that are intended to be rack stable frequently require more nitrates and a more mind boggling drying process that the general individual most likely won't go into, particularly when there's an infrequent auxiliary curing strategy like fixing, aging, or smoking. A few people may do this at home, however it's most ordinarily done at business offices.

Drying – This procedure disposes of all the dampness in a sustenance so that there's no space for any microbial action to move around in the nourishment. This is utilized with a great deal of nourishments and isn't restricted to simply organic products, vegetables, or meats, it's additionally utilized on nuts, grains, vegetables, and fish, among different sustenances. There are various alternatives that you can use to dry sustenance, some of them don't require spending any cash, while different choices imply that you get a dehydrator and will utilize that to take out the greater part of the dampness. As a result of the considerable number of alternatives accessible with regards to drying out nourishment, it's unrealistic to cover everything that you can do to dry out sustenances. Data is promptly accessible at neighborhood libraries or on the web.

Dry Salting – This is a sort of maturation or pickling that is normally utilized with meat, vegetables, and fish. Having a high salt fixation counteracts microbial development and looks after freshness. Individuals who know about dry salting regularly say that the nourishment that outcomes from it tastes superior to anything its canned or solidified partners. This more established strategy for conservation was brought once again into design amid the World Wars to monitor glass, tin, and fuel.

Aging – keeping in mind the end goal to get out perilous bugs, individuals empower the development of "good" microorganisms to avoid nourishment deterioration. This is to a great degree normal, you'll discover this with yogurt, wine, lager, and sauerkraut. As depicted over, the whole purpose of this kind of conservation is to advance the development of good microscopic organisms, and should be possible with no extraordinary hardware. For the most part what necessities to happen (like with cheddar) is the acquaintance of good microscopic organisms with what you're attempting to age. There are various ways this should be possible, and data can be found in libraries or on the web.

Solidifying – This is a standout amongst the most prominent home strategies for sustenance protection. It keeps up the greater part of the supplements that sustenance has and has a genuinely long time span of usability. It might last around an indistinguishable measure of time from canning, and will consume up space in your cooler, yet it is additionally amazingly simple to do. You should simply slice up whatever you're attempting to safeguard and place it in the cooler, more often than not on a sheet plate for a vegetable or an organic product. Ensure that your cooler goes the distance down to 0°F in light of the fact that it may not solidify legitimately in a hotter cooler. Once the sustenance is solidified, make a point to store in a hermetically sealed pack to ensure nothing gets into the nourishment.

Warming – This follows in a similar mentality of bubbling, however doesn't convey sustenance up to the bubbling temperature.

Jellying – all together for this strategy to be done legitimately, the nourishment needs to finish its cooking procedure by winding up in a strong gel. This strategy incorporates utilizing either agar, arrowroot flour, maize flour, or gelatin to make that strong gel. This is a to a great degree prominent path for nourishment to be served in a few zones of the world.

Jugging – Often, the sustenance that leaves this technique winds up in a kind of jam. The way this is done is by taking meat and stewing it in a kind of ceramic container or a meal dish. The meat is cut up and cooked with salt water or sauce in the firmly fixed container, with the likelihood of red wine or creature blood being added to the dish. Until the mid-1900s, this was a famous approach to store meats.

Lye – This makes sustenance excessively salty for microscopic organisms, making it impossible to develop by bringing the soluble level up in the nourishment. This is a technique that is falling marginally out of support as it can be to a great degree hazardous to work with.

Pickling – Pickles are a standout amongst the most widely recognized cases of pickling. So as to do this, you absorb nourishment some kind of corrosive, similar to vinegar, or liquor or salt. Pickling is genuinely simple to do, however can be risky if it's readied severely or if the pickles are held at room temperature. Regularly pickling is joined with maturation, canning, or straightforward refrigeration. Formulas are effectively discovered on the web or in cookbooks.

Fixing – This strategy doesn't totally stop the deterioration of nourishment. Regularly, this strategy is complimentary with different techniques, more often than not with drying or solidifying. This is a to a great degree simple technique for individuals to use at home, as home vacuum sealants are genuinely modest for individuals to purchase. Before purchasing a home vacuum, do research to ensure that it addresses your issues.

Smoking – Often finished with curing, smoking is a complimentary procedure that is said to enhance the flavor and appearance of the sustenance while periodically going about as a drying specialist. In a home domain, there's more flavor and appearance than real conservation, however the nourishment tends to become malodorous or mildew covered or at an extensively bring down rate.

Sugaring – Instead of utilizing salt, a few sustenances are put away in sugar. This most ordinarily happens with organic product being put away in nectar. In a few zones where there isn't sufficient sun to adequately dry sustenance, sugar was utilized. Organic product would be warmed with the sugar, which would get dried out the foods grown from the ground it alright for individuals to eat after a long stockpiling period. There are two or three noteworthy strategies that go into this: one route is to put the natural product in sugar syrup (like nectar), another future to take shape the sugar on the organic product, which would then harden, making something like a candy-coated peel.

There are various different techniques that individuals use to safeguard their nourishments, yet regularly, they fall some place into what we have effectively canvassed in this section or are utilized as a part of business canning or conservation organizations and aren't utilized by home preservers. In case you're interested about alternate techniques, Wikipedia gives a rundown of regular safeguarding strategies.

Conclusion

There are various canning and protection strategies that you can do at home (in case you're not as of now doing them) and some ways that you can do them. A greater part of this book has been spent talking about canning and what you'll have to do keeping in mind the end goal to can. This was done in light of the fact that canning is a standout amongst the most prevalent home protection strategies that individuals can do all alone.

With the ascent of home planting and homestead to-table eating, this book will help you to make sense of what techniques for safeguarding will work best with the nourishment that you're attempting to make last. Canning will help this, as will cooling, jellying, and cellaring, alongside the various techniques.

These techniques will likewise help you to spare cash during the time as they elevate extending nourishment to last out of season consistently. The nourishment that you protect, when safeguarded effectively, will last through the following year and will empower you to purchase a greater amount of the sustenance that you like when it's in season and less expensive. The cycle can be rehashed a seemingly endless amount of time.

This likewise implies the materials that you utilize can regularly be utilized from year to year with a negligible utilization of purchasing new materials. For canning, you should purchase new tops, however that is an insignificant cost in the general comprehension of the amount you spare by reusing a dominant part of your materials. Different strategies for protection additionally have low expenses and high reserve funds, yet you have to comprehend what you're searching for so as to expand your cash.

Formulas are discovered effortlessly on the web, yet ensure that you're utilizing more advanced formulas, particularly with regards to canning for your own particular wellbeing. Botulism is not something that you ought to try and endeavor to mess around with, and a ton of old canning formulas don't have a clue about the breaking point that you have to keep the nourishment at or for to what extent. Some great assets to use for canning formulas incorporate the Ball site and the National Center for Home Preservation. Cookbooks with tried formulas are likewise a decent wellspring of data, however you must be to a great degree watchful and ensure that the cookbook is avant-garde. Various other protection strategies likewise have formulas accessible on the web, simply make a point to check the technique and ensure that it won't make you or your family wiped out.

Ideally, this book has given you a few thoughts on protection and how it can be utilized to extend a dollar in a family that might be tight with cash. Canning is a to a great degree prevalent strategy for conservation, and there are various different less mainstream sorts of safeguarding that are recorded in this book. Ideally, you have some smart thoughts and a heading to go in with regards to home protectio

Resources

Barksdale, Nate. "What It Says on the Tin: A Brief History of Canned Food."*History.com.* A&E Television Networks, 22 Aug. 2014. Web. 09 Sept. 2016.

"Canning Basics For Preserving Food." *Canning Basics For Preserving Food.* N.p., 2008. Web. 10 Sept. 2016.

"Canning." *Wikipedia.* The Wikipedia Foundation, n.d. Web. 9 Sept. 2016.

Colon-Singh, Rosey. "How To Preserve Food | Methods And Techniques."*Fine Dining Lovers.* N.p., 31 July 2016. Web. 10 Sept. 2016.

Esther. "The History Of Home Canning." *Off The Grid News.* Off the Grid News, 2012. Web. 09 Sept. 2016.

Ewald, Jonathan. "What Is Canning and What Are the Benefits?" *Life Health Network.* Life and Health Network, 07 Aug. 2014. Web. 09 Sept. 2016.

"Food Preservation." *Wikipedia.* Wikimedia Foundation, n.d. Web. 10 Sept. 2016.

"Getting Started." *Canning 101.* Hearthmark LLC, n.d. Web. 10 Sept. 2016.

Canning and Preserving

"Home Canning and Botulism." *Centers for Disease Control and Prevention*. Centers for Disease Control and Prevention, 13 June 2016. Web. 09 Sept. 2016.

McClellan, Marisa. "A Beginner's Guide to Canning." *Serious Eats: The Destination for Delicious*. Serious Eats Inc., 29 Feb. 2012. Web. 09 Sept. 2016.

"National Center for Home Food Preservation." *National Center for Home Food Preservation*. N.p., n.d. Web. 10 Sept. 2016.

"An Overview of 10 Home Food Preservation Methods from Ancient to Modern." *The Home Preserving Bible*. N.p., n.d. Web. 10 Sept. 2016.

"The Pros and Cons of Eating Canned Food." *The Alternative Daily*. N.p., 2016. Web. 09 Sept. 2016.

Roche, Brenda. "Home Preserved Foods: Nutrition Friend or Foe?" *ANR Blogs*. University of California, n.d. Web. 09 Sept. 2016.

Stone, Jerry James. "How Canning Was Invented, and How It Changed the Way We Eat - The 5 Greatest Breakthroughs in Food Science." *The Kitchn*. Kitchn, 13 Apr. 2015. Web. 09 Sept. 2016.